The Wealthy Reflexologist

How to Make Over

$100,000 a Year

With Reflexology

By Lauren Slade and Jack Marriott

Published by JL Marriott Publishing

D1593346

Copyright Notice

To our Moms Isabella and Mary
for your inspiration

Contents

Introduction

Anyone who has experienced a basic foot massage knows how relaxing it can be. The rhythmic kneading of feet releases tension, stress and can even relieve migraine headaches and back pain.

How is it that a normal foot massage can do all that – and more? Actually, massaging your feet is a form of Reflexology.

The theory behind this holistic healing art is that the feet have certain points (or triggers) that directly link to the body's various organs. When applying direct pressure to those points, muscles relax, blood circulation is highly improved and the body's immune system reacts by improving your overall condition.

The hands and ears can also improve certain conditions when an experienced Reflexologist applies pressure to related points. Reflexology has been used for centuries in Eastern-style medicine, but is only now making its way to serious consideration in Western medicine methods.

Anyone Can Learn Reflexology

Anyone can learn Reflexology techniques to practice on themselves, friends or family members. There are many online classes available, and you might also find one at your local community college or health care facility.

If you're looking for an experienced Reflexologist, search online for those who are available in your area. Most will have websites where you can learn more about the person and the services they offer – including prices.

The number of people wanting to become a Reflexologist has multiplied and is now one of the top five career options in the holistic health field. The trend toward holistic medicine as a career is a reflection of many problems in traditional health care practices.

High cost of traditional health care is one problem, and more people want permanent answers to their health problems rather than the quick fixes of surgery or pills to mask a larger problem.

If you're thinking of pursuing a career in Reflexology, look for a program that takes a deeper look at the connection between the reflex trigger points and a holistic lifestyle with proper nutrition, and exercise. It's also important to find a school or program that teaches ethics, professionalism, and how to manage the financial aspect of running a Reflexology business.

This book, "The Wealthy Reflexologist" or "How to Make Over $100,000 a Year with Reflexology," will provide some important information about how to get started in your business as a Reflexologist – and how to turn it into a stellar financial success!

Chapter 1 – Create the Mindset for Success

We don't always see the big picture of success no matter what our career. Many times, those in the holistic healing professions limit their practice and don't think outside the box as to what *could* be if they cultivated the multitude of areas where their profession could flourish. Reflexology professionals often see themselves as healers, but don't understand or know how to go about running their profession as a business.

To create a mindset for success, you must first look at the art of Reflexology as a profession worthy of recognition – especially financial recognition. Reflexology is a profession that is fast becoming highly recognized for the science of healing that it brings to individuals. Now is the time to seize the opportunity of success that recognition brings.

As Reflexologists, we already have the mindset of helping people. In fact, most of us are driven to help others heal and are proud of the knowledge we possess to do that. Sometimes, we're so intense on helping others that we forego the fees that other types of practitioners charge – so that **everyone** can experience our passion -- and end up never achieving financial success.

It's as if charging a fee for healing somehow puts a price on our internal belief system – that everyone should be free of pain. We're often oblivious to rules of financial success, believing instead that service to others is the top priority and financial rewards aren't the reason we entered the profession in the first place.

That said, it's also important, as a fellow Reflexologist, to maintain and boost the credibility of Reflexology as a healing modality. This is accomplished in part by charging fees that are comparable to other healing professions.

Financial success is not only important to our own well-being, but imperative when building an image that coincides with the healing power that we offer. If we can't accomplish this, it may mean the downfall of our businesses. An altruistic attitude won't pay the bills and our businesses may suffer if we can't make financial success a reality.

Many are content to bring in a nice yearly income of $50,000 per year. But what if we could show you a way to double that figure? $100,000 per year and more is at your fingertips if you'll make up your mind to follow the path to success. You have it in your power to be financially successful and help others beyond your expectations if you'll put this plan into action.

The result of business failure could mean the end to your being able to help others. We want you to succeed and share your skills and abilities with others. To be successful you want to develop both your Reflexology skills and knowledge as well as your business and success mindset. By developing business acumen and using your talents to achieve success, you'll be doing yourself a big favour – and encouraging others to do the same by setting an example.

Attitude Makes a Huge Difference

Of all the various types of businesses, a positive attitude is of the utmost importance in alternative health care. When you meet clients as a Reflexologist, your attitude can make the difference in a client leaving with a "can do" mentality or a frown on their face.

You can either build your business or never see that one-time client again.

It's sometimes difficult to maintain a positive attitude when things in your life aren't going your way. During those times, a professional mind set must take over. With that, you'll need to find the strength you need to be responsible for your clients' welfare and ensure that they'll return.

Since Reflexologists come from a place that is all about mind, body and spirit, you also have a responsibility to keep yourself and your mind healthy and positive. No one takes a person seriously who isn't following the path she presents to others. This mindset is one of the most important parts of the successful business you're trying to create.

When you spend your precious time with a client complaining or gossiping about others and generally presenting a negative outlook, the client misses the best part of his or her session – relaxation. The best and most successful reflexologists begin their sessions with words such as, "This is your time and I want you to get the most of it – so just lie back and put everything out of your mind." **Then, be quiet!**

When you come into a session or meet a new client with a self-defeating attitude, it will show and result in a disappointing session with the client. These negative thoughts limit your ability to provide a successful Reflexology session and can make or break your business.

Be honest with yourself. If you find yourself sinking into despair or negativity, take a lesson from your alternative health counterparts. Learn relaxing techniques by developing Yoga deep breathing skills and practice getting rid of negative thoughts the second they enter your mind. And, don't use negative words in your every day speech – even when you're not with a client.

You'll soon find that your business is becoming successful – and your personal life is bound to improve as well.

The Mindset for Financial Success

It's a given that Reflexology professionals are motivated to help others. Many are content to settle for low fees because they want everyone to have access to the healing powers they possess.

Promotions and discounts can provide people with a way to get the benefits of Reflexology without spending a lot of money. But, for the most part, your hourly fees should be set to the standards of other health care professionals.

In the beginning, be sure that your fees are comparable to other Reflexologists in the area and that they're a reflection of your experience, reputation and skill level. If you discover that you're charging too much (or too little), adjust your fees as needed.

When you begin to consider yourself a health care professional and open your own business, you can justify charging higher fees for your services. And, when you offer a wide range of Reflexology techniques (not just foot Reflexology) and hire others with similar skills to expand your business, you'll be surprised at how people are willing to pay for the quality of service received.

You'll reach that $100,000 per year goal before you know it and can grow your business according to your own interests.

Reflexologists are in demand! Reflexologists are earning $50 - $100 per hour in private practice. A recent poll of 1,401 visitors to my website, said that 54.53% would be willing to pay between $50 and $100 for a Reflexology session with 3% willing to pay more than $100 dollars for an hour of relaxation heaven.

How does that translate into business income for you? Let's do some simple math...

If you were to work on 3 clients per day and let's take an average of $75 per session – that is $225 per day. If you work only five days a week that is $1,125 per week, so per year that works out to $58, 500 per year. – That is only working 3 actual hours per day plus some set up time. If you decided to take up to 6 clients a day – that is $117,000 per year.

Depending on your definition of rich, that is either a good annual income or a healthy supplement to your everyday living expenses. And we haven't even discussed all the little extras that you can add into your Reflexology practice to earn even more!

Day to day expenses of a Reflexology business are quite small depending on where you decide to work, but if you work from home, and use the internet for advertising, your overhead costs are quite minimal.

We will discuss the many varied aspects of how and where to obtain these clients throughout this book.

A poll for the BBC in Britain indicated that 21% (or 1 in 5) of Britons have used a complementary medicine or therapy in the last year - double the number found to be using them in a similar survey six years ago.

The majority of people said the main reason they used alternative medicine was because it worked for them, but other reasons included that it was relaxing and that it helped prevent illness. One in ten Brits was referred to an alternative therapist by their medical doctor.

Do you know that health spas charge as much as $250 for one Reflexology session? Do you know why they charge that amount of money? Because they have customers who are willing to pay handsomely for the benefits to their health, and as the BBC survey said, customers find it a relaxing experience that can also help prevent illness.

Envisioning Financial Success

Every person who has achieved financial success has first had a vision of what it would look and feel like. Your vision may include being your own boss, and having your own space where you train and keep employees to expand your business.

Having a vision of the space you would create and how you would look within that space is very important to staying focused on what's important to you. A vision board is a great way to make sure that vision is in front of you at all times.

For example, envision the way you would look in your business environment. Look for pictures in magazines and brochures about how you would appear as a successful Reflexologist. Visualize the finest details of your practice, including the comfortable and neat clothes you'd wear – perhaps a jacket with the name of your business embroidered on it.

Have a vision about how the inside of your business space would look when your clients come in. Even if it's a room in your home, picture it as spotlessly clean and inviting. What equipment would you have in the room? Perhaps a massage table or recliner. Soft music playing in the background and scented candles placed strategically around the room can be part of the overall picture.

What would you do if you were making $100,000+ per year as a successful Reflexology business? You may want to pin vacation ideas on your vision board. Is your dream to own a sports car? Find the one you want and pin that on the board too.

There's no end to what you can imagine with a vision board. Thousands have used this method to create success in their lives – both financial and personal.

Keep Them Coming Back

If you're going to achieve financial success in Reflexology, you're going to have to develop a mindset to keep clients returning on a regular basis. You have your Reflexology certification and a business plan – now, you must work on marketing your business and keep the clients returning and spreading news about your business.

Your mindset has everything to do with building a clientele. Think beyond the box – like offering a product line that will increase your "reach" to clients. You don't need to know everything about Reflexology, but you should be continually learning. You'll then be able to talk to your clients about new techniques to help them.

There are people out there who desperately need your services. Don't be afraid to talk to people about what you can offer them. Also, listen to what your clients – and others you talk to – say so that you can give them exactly what they want.

Set a realistic price according to your experience and expertise. Knowing that your clients are not under- or over- paying for your services is a good way to keep you feeling good about yourself and the services you offer.

Have a space to call your own. Even if it's only a separate room in your home, designating a space of your own will help you realize that you're running a business and have an obligation to your clients to run it to the best of your ability.

Believe in yourself. That is perhaps the most important way to keep your mindset positive and build your business successfully. Let people, especially clients, know that you're proud of what you do and that their feedback is invaluable to you to make sure you're meeting their needs.

Find ways to keep yourself motivated. It's quite normal to get up some mornings and feel that you just can't be positive or successful in treating your clients. The "karma" just isn't there.

Discover what keeps you motivated and frees your mind from the constrictions of self-doubt and practice it 24/7 – not only when you're feeling down in the dumps. It's a daily challenge to reprogram your mind if you want to drink from the well of creativity and abundance in your life.

Develop a "prosperity" mindset. It will help you on your path to success and help you through any challenges you might face along the way. Developing a prosperity mindset means that you must have a plan (financial and personal) and stick to it.

Give 110% of yourself in all that you do. Setting up a business is challenging and you're bound to experience some setbacks, but if your mindset is tuned in to success, you'll overcome those obstacles and success will be yours!

Chapter 2 -
Financial Success as a
Reflexologist

Everyone who has achieved financial success has first developed a plan to get there. Nothing happens without one. The starting point is to assess the financial situation you're in now. Without that knowledge, you're pretty much doomed to fail. With it, you'll be able to visualize a financially successful future and able to jump the hurdles you're sure to face.

After you assess your current financial situation, it's time to develop a plan of success. This may mean that you have to face problems, learn from them, adapt and then solve them so that you can achieve all your goals and make your dreams a reality.

The vision you have of your Reflexology business can be your greatest motivator. You'll gain energy and a fervent desire to make success happen with a clear vision of success and how it looks. Channelling your vision into the direction it needs to travel will help you stay focused and win any challenges that come your way.

You may imagine that owning your own Reflexology business and being your own boss are the perfect factors in living a happy and rewarding life. It can be the fulfilment of a dream – but not based on how great you are at Reflexology. The success of your business is going to depend on how well you manage it.

Owning and managing your own business isn't a free pass to leave whenever you want and put a "Closed" sign on the door and go shopping or out to lunch. Maintaining a professional image is important to your lasting success. Establish a dedicated space for your new practice and keep regular hours just like any business.

The more professional you and your business appear to others, the more likely your business is to grow and become a financial success. It may take a while to build your Reflexology business to the point that you have a steady stream of clients, but it will happen if you have a business plan and carry it out.

Having a well-thought out plan and managing your business correctly are keys to reaching success. Write down your plan for daily, weekly, monthly, short-term and long-term goals and revisit it often to be sure you're on the right track. If you see something isn't working, now is the perfect time to revise.

Treat your business professionally and get the word out by joining (and being active in) organizations such as your local Chamber of Commerce. Not only will your business get a boost from the visibility, but you'll meet people who can share their business knowledge and could become your clients.

Difference Between Advertising & Marketing

Knowing every aspect of what you'll need to run a successful Reflexology business includes understanding the difference between advertising and marketing your business. Most people confuse the two, but some basic knowledge will help you with your business plan.

Basically, the definition of advertising is a "non-personal announcement of your products and services through an identified platform or sponsor to an existing audience." Marketing is defined as "the process of producing a strategy and plan which is methodically implemented."

The aim of marketing your business is "to systematically plan and put into place the price promotion, services and distribution to create and maintain relationships that will deliver your organizational and individual objectives – i.e., bringing buyers and sellers together for an exchange of products or services."

You can combine the two methods to create a successful strategy of getting the word out about your business – and, making sure you're expressing what you want people to know about you and Reflexology.

Tips & Tactics to Spread the Word

Any successful business must have marketing strategies. It's not enough to tell your friends and family that you can now practice Reflexology and expect them to get the word out. You must reach others outside your social and family circle.

The correct Reflexology marketing techniques can add real value and visibility to your business and help you achieve ultimate financial success. Marketing techniques aren't usually thought of by Reflexologists when they begin their practices, so learning about them and which are best for you is a must.

Reflexology is a "quiet" business and various methods of communication aren't something that most Reflexologists are familiar with. They may communicate successfully with clients, friends and family on a personal basis, but depend on business cards, yellow page ads and word of mouth to increase their client base.

As part of your Reflexology business plan, and marketing strategy, you should also include communication with others outside your comfort zone. For example, resolve to meet at least ten people every day with the sole purpose of promoting your business. Make personal contact with them, offer a business card or brochure and be enthusiastic.

When you meet people for the first time, the usual conversation that comes up in the first few minutes is, "What do you do?" When you say, "I'm a Reflexologist," that statement will naturally open the door to how it works, where you practice, and you can also get in to all the maladies that Reflexology may be able to 'help fix.'

Stress is the number one complaint among today's harried population. Stress is the cause of many diseases and even a shortened life span.

The American Institute of Stress has determined that stress costs businesses nearly $300 billion annually – which works out to be approximately $7,500 per employee.

Talk about how Reflexology can help to relieve stress. Nine out of ten people will be extremely interested and some may want to give it a try.

Always try and get the other person's name and email address. Have a pen and one of your business cards on hand and let them write the information on the back. Also, give them one of your cards to keep.

Even if only one in ten of the people you meet on a daily basis calls and becomes a client – think of how that could boost your yearly income! You may not think of your Reflexology profession as one that requires "meeting and greeting," but if you don't get the word out on a personal level, you could be missing the angle that could take you to that target number of $100,000 per year.

Every time you secure a new client, be sure to provide them with cards and brochures when they leave and ask them to pass them out to people they know. If you don't do that, you're missing out on one of the best ways to promote your business – word-of-mouth from people who have actually benefited from your practice.

Marketing Tools to Grow Your Business

You may not have chosen the profession of Reflexology to learn marketing, but marketing your business is the key to growing and getting the most satisfaction – both financially and personally.

Before you haphazardly begin to use marketing tools to create interest in your business, sit down and have a plan in mind. Write down what your objectives are – what you want to accomplish from the methods you choose.

The marketing tools you use to grow your client base need to convince them that you provide value and skill for the fees you charge. Aside from making a point to meet people and tell them about yourself and be sure you're in the yellow pages of the phone book, there are several other methods that can help get your name to the public and generate interest.

Here are a few resources you can choose from to get the word out about you and your business:

⇨ Website.

⇨ Local advertising, including store windows, newspapers, local magazines and bulletin boards.

⇨ Online blogs. Create your own blog and have a link to your website.

⇨ Flyers. Hire high schoolers or other young people looking for work to hand them out.

⇨ Third party websites. Many social websites let you link your web page to posted comments or photos you've made.

⇨ Cost per click advertisements. This is called "search engine marketing," and occurs when users click on to your website. You pay a nominal fee for each click, but it's a great way to drive people to your website.

Don't limit your advertising and marketing efforts to only one method. It will limit your growth and completely disregard other sectors that you could be tapping in to for more business.

Try several marketing and advertising methods to see which work best in your area. You'll quickly notice those that become less effective and can weed them out accordingly.

A brochure that enthusiastically describes you and your work is a great marketing tool for Reflexologists. Before you decide on content and design, find and gather as many brochures from other healers as you can. Alternative book stores and health food stores are great places to find a wide variety of these brochures.

Brochures must address the needs and wants of future clients. Do you know the person who created the brochure you picked up? Is that Reflexologist successful? The brochure should immediately grab the attention of the average person by giving them something they want or need.

The truth is, many people don't understand or know what Reflexology can do for them, so if you're trying to pique their interest by telling them how it works, they probably won't be interested. They want to know specifics about how it can help them – personally. They want to know the answer to the age old question, "What's In It For Me?"

People aren't willing to 'buy' Reflexology from you, but they'll be more than willing to purchase a sure-fired stress reliever, and/or a cure for certain ailments such as frayed nerves, pain and lack of flexibility. It's all about how you can make them feel.

If you design your brochures with the idea of promoting the fact that you can actually help a person to feel better, you'll get much more attention than explaining how Reflexology works and that you're really good at it.

Most people today simply don't feel as good as they'd like. And, most would pay almost any amount of money to feel better - to be without the aches, pains, stress and chronic depression that plagues them on a daily basis.

We now know that stress can certainly lead to chronic diseases and other problems, so the world is full of ideas on how to "beat stress." Massage, yoga and even de-stressors such as electric neck and foot massagers are becoming popular ways that people are attempting to reduce the stress factors and results in their lives.

But, so many still don't know about the advantages of Reflexology. Your brochures and any other way you choose to communicate with others should always state what you can do for them and how the techniques that you know and are good at can change their lives. Oh–, and they'll really enjoy it too.

The phone can also be a marketing tool if you know how to use it. Make it part of your practice to call clients the day after a Reflexology session and ask them how they're feeling and how they would rate the session as to how much better it made them feel.

If you don't yet have an Internet website, have one designed. Then, be sure you put the site on your business cards and brochures. It might cost a little money to have a site professionally designed, but it will pay off in the long run. Look at other Reflexologists' websites and get some ideas from those that appeal to you.

You may want to consider running a 'special' from time to time. One way this can be accomplished is to package several sessions for one price. Take a significant amount off the total price – or give a session free if they purchase five at once. This can serve to bring clients in on a regular basis, and keep them coming long after the special has passed.

As Reflexologists, we're trained to improve and heal the mind, body and spirit. You'll have more clients than you can manage if you can effectively convince them that they need you.

Online Advertising for Bigger Profits

There are a number of free places online where you can list your practice. Free online directories are a great source for getting the word out. Since most people are using online resources rather than phone directories or other means to find products and services, it makes good sense to list your business with these online directories.

Free online directories are great, but if you really want to get the word out quickly about your business, the Internet also offers "Paid for Directories," where you pay a fee to ensure high traffic to your site.

Your ad, containing a link to your website, will be placed in the directory of a third party website that may or may not be seen by a large audience. It's recommended that you research online for the most advantageous site to place information about your practice to ensure success.

For example, you wouldn't place an ad for your business in Toronto or New York City on a rural road in Saskatchewan or Texas. It's the same with placing an ad online. Just be sure that it's going to be seen by those in your area and by those who are interested in holistic healing methods and might use your service.

Also pay attention to the amount of space you're allotted to describe your business and the art of Reflexology – how it can help others to relieve stress, pain and other mental conditions.

You'll want your site to look professional and not crowded with information, but yet fully describing all of the services that you offer.

Your best online advertising can come from your own website. You may want to consider a professional web designer to set it up for you to be sure it looks attractive and is working properly.

A website gives you the ability to advertise 24/7. It's always available for those who want more information or to call you to make an appointment.

Today, people who are looking for information on your business assume that you have a website. If you don't have a working website for your Reflexology business, people searching for you might think you're not established properly, are new or that you're not insured, among other things.

Another reason to have a website is that people are looking for as much information as they can gather before they make a decision about alternative medical and complementary therapy techniques. Some who have never tried it are curious and want to know more about it. Your website can provide them with the information they're seeking, thus establishing you as a valuable and trustworthy provider.

Create a website that thoroughly explains your services, and be sure to include testimonials from those who have experienced relief from Reflexology treatments. Don't make the site boring, but do briefly include some statistics about how Reflexology helps relieve stress, migraines, back pain, tension and much more. Remember, your potential clients want to know what's in it for them – stress the benefits of Reflexology and your services.

Your clients can also use your site to contact you about information they need or to ask you to call them. Finding you in the phone book might mean that they forget to call – or worse, call someone else if you're not available.

There are great website services that are designed professionally and that specialize in holistic therapists. Some even offer discounts if you're new and have never used their services before. For affordable website solutions refer to the resource section at the back of this book.

Determine Your Advertising Budget

You'll want to get the word out as best you can, but you can spend too much on an advertising budget and still not attract clients. You may be targeting the wrong group(s). So, it's not actually the amount of money you spend on advertising, but the value you get for your money.

On the other hand, you might spend a lower amount on an advertising method that gets you very little success for the money, while spending a larger amount on a more effective advertising method might convert to gaining more clients.

You certainly don't want to waste money in advertising costs, so you must do your research very carefully and wisely choose an advertising venue that will give you the best bang for the buck.

The main thing you'll need to consider in determining your advertising budget is where your customers will come from. You may not be able to determine this until you try a few methods of advertising, but if you keep a chart of places you advertise and then ask inquiring clients where they got your number; you'll soon see where your ads are making the most impact.

If you've got a website up and running, you can use an 'analytics package' to track your clients and see which pages on your website is getting the most views. The one we recommend is "Google Analytics." It's completely free and does a great job of tracking your online hits.

Understanding Your Target Market

Crafting a financially successful business plan means that you must understand who you're targeting your Reflexology services to. Who are your potential clients? Understanding the demographics of your area helps and also determines your advertising and marketing locales.

Marketers understand that not every brochure or advertisement will catch everyone's attention, and online marketing is different because clients find you – not the other way around. But you still need to advertise on sites that give you the most exposure to the clientele you're seeking to attract.

The lines between marketing "categories" sometimes blur. For example, you can't expect every "senior" to be interested in Reflexology treatments and you also can't expect every teenager to dismiss it.

Perhaps in the past you may have been able to base your targeting on income, ethnicity, education or gender, however in today's fast paced, ever changing world, that is no longer possible. Personalization is one way to market your services. By letting them know that you are thinking of each perspective client's lifestyle and what they need as individuals, you'll speak to their inner being and have much more success.

For example, many marketers in the past have dismissed the baby boomers after age 50. Today, we know they have a strong buying power and influence, and we also know that they're grasping alternative medicine as an answer to high medical costs and increasing aches and pains as they age.

Gen I and Gen Y generations are savvy about finding services on the computer, and are much more accepting of new technology that promises relief from tension and stress. Mostly, they're known for thinking outside the box, so these groups of people might be very responsive to your Reflexology advertising and marketing campaigns – especially online marketing.

Gen Xers came after the baby boomer generation and they can be classified as at the peak of their earning power. Born between 1965 and 1975, this generation is tech-savvy. They value education and new health techniques. They also like to save money when they can and want to know that the services you're offering are good values.

Often overlooked in many marketing strategies is The Greatest Generation – born between 1909 and 1945. But this group is living longer that ever and tends to value services such as Reflexology because it can relieve pain and preserve health.

Keep in mind the current state of the economy. When you have a well-defined target market for your services, study how your geographic area has been affected. Some parts of the country have been affected more than others, and you should base your fees partly on that consideration.

Focusing your marketing budget with a message that targets certain areas and people is necessary to make the most of your money. Periodically - look over your current customer base. Where are most of your clients coming from and what are their concerns?

Some other factors to consider when you're deciding on a target market for Reflexology services are:

- Can they afford your services?

- What drives your target market into decision making?

- Is the area large enough to support your services?

An abundance of valuable information can be found by researching online. Other Reflexologists are also great resources – and recent demographic surveys can also be a big help. Remember to make good use of the Internet when deciding who and where your target market is.

Targeting your clientele for a successful marketing campaign can be very useful – but don't over-think the strategy. In an area such as Reflexology, you'll have a wider market than you could ever expect, and gather clients from all areas and personality types.

Chapter 3 - The Bones of a Successful Reflexology Business

The foundation (or bones) of any successful business depends on how well you treat your business within – just like the bones within your body. If you don't exercise and eat the right foods for good bone health, you could be subjected to diseases such as Osteoporosis and Arthritis. The foundation of a business will also crumble if you don't take the time and effort to make sure the bones are strong.

Self-management is the key strategy that will ensure your Reflexology business is a successful one. If you can't manage yourself and your time, there's very little hope that you'll be able to manage a successful business.

Whatever you desire in life can be achieved with the proper self-management techniques. That means directing your life like you were a director of an epic movie – determining each twist and turn that your life and your business will take to lead it to a "happy" ending.

Do you need to increase you client base? Then, you have to find a way to meet more people and to get the word out about your business. How about the financial end of your Reflexology business? Perhaps you need to seek the advice of a professional financial planner to help you meet your goals and fulfil your desires.

But no one is going to know how to successfully run your life except you. Taking personal responsibility for yourself and your actions, taking control of your time, education and keeping yourself in tune and dedicated to self-improvement are just a few of the elements involved in becoming and remaining successful.

Any business takes time to build. You're going to have some hurdles you never dreamed of facing and make mistakes as well as achieve triumphs. One of the advantages you have over others just starting out in business is that Reflexology and other alternative healing methods are booming.

More people are becoming savvy about the benefits of alternative medicine – and especially Reflexology. With the high costs of insurance and other, traditional health care costs, people are seeking alternative medical treatments – and that means your Reflexology business is sure to grow in the years to come.

It takes time to build your clientele, but if you work at it diligently and make a name for yourself in your area, you'll soon be able to expand and offer a variety of services by other professionals.

You Are a Professional

Do anything and everything it takes to know your business inside and out. When a client asks you a question, you want to be able to address it with knowledge and confidence. That alone will set you up as a professional to your clients. Exuding confidence and professionalism will also help your mindset about charging a realistic fee.

Offer professional cards, brochures and other advertising media that expressly targets your clientele. For example, if you want to specialize in relieving stress, make that a prominent factor in your advertising material.

You should always be ethical – and that means not gossiping or tearing down another Reflexologist's business or techniques. Your clients want peace when they come to you and not to feel uncomfortable about your remarks about others.

Offering a variety of services to your clients is also a way to build your professionalism – and increase your financial worth. Consider hiring or contracting with other service professionals such as massage therapists, reiki practitioners or acupuncturists to broaden your practice.

A lot of Reflexology professionals only offer foot Reflexology, but you can also train for or hire others who are trained in hand, ear, meridian, maternity and facial Reflexology. These additional services are growing in popularity at the same level as the foot Reflexology techniques, and they will offer a good variety to your clients – who will pass the word along to others.

Setting yourself up as a professional in your field also means that you should look the part. Highly successful salons and Reflexology and other massage businesses have a dress code that looks professional and is comfortable to wear. Your healing space should also have professional – and clean – equipment.

Communicating With Your Clients

Another key to building and maintaining your Reflexology business from the inside is successful communicating with your clients. For example, while you shouldn't chat continuously during a session, it's perfectly okay to ask how he or she is feeling during the middle of the treatment.

Truly listen to your clients. Invite them to be completely honest about the level of treatment they're receiving by letting you know if what you're doing hurts or is uncomfortable or if they'd prefer more or less pressure in some areas than others.

They'll leave the session realizing that you have their well-being in mind and so relaxed and stress-free afterward that they'll be anxious to make another appointment – the sooner the better.

Calling your customer a day or two after the session and asking for an evaluation is a great way to let them know that you care about the experience they had and to know if you're on the right track to building your client base.

One unique way of communicating with clients is to provide a caring and relaxing environment. Your treatment surroundings can impress or turn off your customers. Even though you might give the best Reflexology treatment in town, you won't become successful if your environment is lacking.

Some Reflexologists work out of their homes in the beginning. If your home is your setting, be sure you have a space designated especially for your clients – free from clutter such as toys, dirty clothes and other turn-offs. Always maintain a pristine treatment area.

Some Reflexologists add soft music (and play it at a low volume), scented candles and oils. Clean, warm blankets will help to create the relaxing mood you're striving for and your clients will feel pampered and special. However, be really aware of possible allergies to any perfumes or oils you may use, and always check with your clients prior to them arriving in your clinic room. If the area is filled with strong scents, a sensitive client may leave and never return!

Correctly setting and communicating your hours of operation to your clients is also important to send a message that you're appreciative of their time and efforts to seek you out and spend time and money for their treatments.

When setting hours of operation, keep in mind that the more flexible you are, the more clients will find your services appealing. Everyone has a hectic schedule now and if you have a typical 9 to 5 mentality, your business growth may be limited.

If a client complains about a scheduling problem, try to accommodate them. You may need to work nights or even make house calls, but if you're serious about growing your business, you'll soon be reaping the results of your flexibility.

Some Reflexologists conduct "self-help seminars" for their clients that teach them how to perform some of the techniques that might help them relieve chronic pain or soreness. Take some additional training so you can offer complimentary services. For example, you might want to offer aromatherapy or herbal recipes. Broadening your services offers more value to your clients and can make your practice more desirable.

Reflexology Business In Your Home

Most Reflexologists who are new to the business begin their careers either in a spa or start their own at-home Reflexology space. They begin experimenting with techniques with family members and friends to learn what works and what doesn't.

As you develop your brochures and get the word out about your new career, you'll be building a clientele that will likely follow you when you decide to expand to a space outside your home.

The clientele will eventually spread from a family and friends base to people outside your sphere. It's the way that many stay at home moms who decided to study and become certified as Reflexologists have found lucrative incomes to supplement household finances.

Many have studied Reflexology as a way to manage their own or a family member's pain from an injury or disease. One special Reflexologist began studying Reflexology to be able to manage their son's behaviour issues that resulted from a brain injury. Eventually, she and another mother founded a rehabilitation centre for studies in neurological development. The centre uses Reflexology successfully in the programs taught and practiced there.

If you do choose to begin your Reflexology business in your home, be sure to check with your city or town licensing department to see if there are limits to the types of businesses you can open in your home.

No matter how you get in to the study and practice of Reflexology and no matter where you choose to have your space, it's a wonderful way to gradually ease into a lucrative career and grow it to an incredible and rewarding business.

Mobile Reflexology Services

Expanding your Reflexology business can include mobile services – especially if you're just starting out in the field and need to build a client base. There are many areas that you might extend your services to, including:

Cosmetic Salons – These types of salons are popping up all over and most would jump at the chance to expand their business by offering Reflexology services. They usually offer various facial cleanses and perhaps makeup application and/or classes. Forging an alliance with one or more of these salons is a good way for you both to extend your businesses to a variety of clientele. You can use a space in their salon (be sure it meets your standards) and call you or have the client call you for an appointment. It's a win-win alliance.

Hair Salons – Once again, these salons may not have need for a full time Reflexologist, but would enjoy using your mobile services to increase their clientele and their money-making abilities.

Hospices and Nursing Homes – Expanding your Reflexology services to include visiting hospice and nursing homes would be an ideal setting for you to help others while expanding your clientele. People who reside in these communities would enjoy and respond positively to the "healing touch" of Reflexology and many have no way to get to a salon or treatment centre. Your mobile Reflexology business would be the answer to many prayers for healing and pain management.

Businesses – More and more businesses are realizing the need to help relieve stress for employees in order to increase productivity. Many businesses offer workout facilities and even pay for the services of a masseuse if requested by employees. Approach businesses as a professional who can provide services that will help relieve stress for employees, increase productivity and promote good will. Have answers ready for questions they might ask and be willing and ready to work with them on hours and availability.

Starting out your Reflexology business by offering mobile services can bring many benefits, including an increase in clientele and a boost to your income. Meet prospective clients armed with carefully designed business cards and brochures that reflect exactly what you offer – and how it can benefit them.

Partnering With Doctors & Hospitals

More doctors and hospitals are realizing the benefits of partnering with Reflexologists and other alternative care practitioners to enhance their own medical therapies. You may want to consider partnering with a doctor or hospital – especially if you're just starting your business and don't have your own space.

Certain types of doctors, such as chiropractors and podiatrists, may especially realize the need for your Reflexology services. Try talking to someone at a holistic health centre about offering your services there if there is one nearby. Local gyms and spas might also be a good place to start your business and have clients come to you.

Also, a doctor and/or hospital may help market your services which can save you a lot on initial start-up costs. If you're partnering with another business, they might dictate the fees you can charge, while others will let you set your own prices.

Besides keeping up with techniques through online or local classes, be sure that you check Reflexology websites often and subscribe to holistic health magazines and newsletters to keep you informed about new trends and tips.

When you make an appointment to speak with a doctor or someone at a holistic care centre, gym or spa about partnering with them and offering your services, be sure that you've got a "speech" prepared.

They'll want to know how much experience you've had, and if you're new, that's not much. Instead of just saying, "None," talk about your volunteer work with non-paying clients, friends and family members that you've helped to relieve aches and pains.

Also, discuss your training and how excited you are to make a difference in people's health experiences. Your enthusiasm is key in getting them to pay attention and offer you a position with their practice or at their place of business.

Ethics of Reflexology

The International Council of Reflexologists commits its members to a Code of Ethic and Practice. It outlines the ethical and professional principles and standards for membership in the organization.

The ICR Code of Ethics is divided into three sections, "Guiding Principles," "Responsibilities to Clients" and "Responsibility Toward the Profession." Among the guiding principles are that each member should "skilfully and caringly practice Reflexology for the benefit of the client."

Among the Responsibilities to Clients section is the edict that "members shall keep full and accurate records while maintaining client confidentiality. "Responsibility Toward the Profession" includes that "a member shall participate in the profession's effort to protect the public from misinformation and inform the public about the benefits of Reflexology.

Ethics should be practiced among every health care profession, whether traditional or alternative medicine. Standards of the profession encompass many aspects of the code of ethics among physicians and other health care providers.

One of the aspects of running a successful Reflexology practice is creating and maintaining a line of trust between you and your clients. That means providing accurate information. If there's something you don't know, either find the answer or refer them to someone else.

All your clients deserve the utmost respect and consideration. Provide a clean and relaxing space for their treatments and interview them each time so that you can get an accurate account of what's going on in their lives and with their bodies.

Only perform the services that you're specifically qualified to perform and never lead the customer astray by offering them information about Reflexology that you're not well-versed in. Also, don't verbally put down any other medical profession or alternative health care technique.

In fact, if they're curious about other techniques to help their situations, get the information for them or lead them to a place where they can find the information themselves.

Never run down another Reflexologist, even if you question his or her techniques. If you're asked a specific question about another in the profession, respectfully decline to answer. You'll gain much respect for not commenting when you have nothing good to say.

When you set up a Reflexology practice with unquestionable ethics, you'll get respect not only from your clients, but also from others in the profession.

Chapter 4 - The Financial Side of Your Reflexology Business

Reflexologists have the reputation of being some of the most gentle and generous people in the world. They're healers – and most aren't in it for the money, but because they have a passion for helping people. They set their fees low and spend more time with clients just to go the extra mile in helping them feel better.

If you are a Reflexologist that has a passion for helping people, and also wants to earn a good income, we have great news for you. There are steps you can take to set up your Reflexology business to become extremely successful and make $100,000 per year, or more, from it.

Setting up your own Reflexology business to be successful includes continuing your education. There are advances being made in this dynamic healing art, and you need to be sure that you're informed.

Find a mentor who has built a successful Reflexology business and pattern your practice from what they've done while developing your own style. Then, become a mentor to other fledgling Reflexologists. You'll be rewarded in countless ways for your generosity and leadership.

Cultivate friendships with colleagues and encourage your group to challenge and motivate each other. You'll be surprised and delighted at how much support you can get from those who think and work in the same line as you. Ideas will flow and you'll learn tricks from them about how to manage finances.

Tips for Setting Up a Financial Plan

Those of us in health and wellness careers often make mistakes that are avoidable if you know about them ahead of time. Here are some tips for ensuring the financial success of your Reflexology business:

Have a carefully thought out business plan. You may need the help of someone who knows how to set up a business, but there are many online courses and help that will get you started, and that may be all you need.

Work on your business acumen as much as learning new healing skills. It may seem boring and mundane, but it's a necessary part of building a successful business. It may help to get the advice of an accountant, especially for taxes.

Have a legal plan in place. You should know exactly what's required for your business to be legitimate. For example, know the legalities involved in setting up a sole proprietorship, LLC or partnership if these plans are necessary for your business.

Research marketing plans of other successful Reflexologists. Look until you find one that's right for you and then set it up to your standards.

Leverage yourself. You can earn more money and make your Reflexology business successful by keeping a product line on hand to sell to customers, making investments (you'll need a professional financial advisor for this) and hiring a staff so that you'll earn a commission on their skills and clients.

Once you have a business plan in place, the nuts and bolts of the actual financial plan should contain three financial statements. These include the income statement, cash flow projection and a balance sheet.

You'll divide your business into two categories – start-up expenses and actual operating expenses.

Here are some start-up expenses that you might need to jot down:

- Furniture and equipment – a rolling stool for you and a recliner and/or massage table for your clients.

- A starting inventory of products and lotions and oils that you'll need.

- Local business licensing and registration fees.

- Rent for space in a building – or determining a space in your home and how much you can deduct in taxes.

- Down payments on utilities for the space you're renting or designating.

- Business computer and software.

- Communication fees and space in local telephone book.

- Brochures and business cards.

Actual operating expenses might look like this:

- Rent and utilities.

- Promotions for your business such as newsletters, ads in local newspapers and flyers.

- Salaries for you and staff (if any).

- Supplies such as cleaning products, towels, etc.

The first step in getting your financial statement ready to go is to estimate the above expenses. Then, multiply that number by six and you'll have a six month estimate of what your Reflexology business will cost. Add that to your start-up expenses and you'll have the complete cost of starting and running your business.

You'll find actual forms online that you can print out and fill in – or you might try software designed to track expenses.

Creating a Cash Flow Projection

This is an important tool for your overall financial plan and one that will help you know when you're spending too much or not enough. It's a pretty simple concept showing what you anticipate the cash flow will be for the future of your business.

The cash flow statement shows the past cash in and cash out of your business. While the cash flow projection statement shows how cash is expected to flow in and out of your business. It can help you make adjustments to your payables and receivables to maintain a positive cash flow.

Later, if you decide to expand the business, and need a loan, a bank will take a careful look at this cash flow projection for proof that your expansion is a good risk for them to take.

You can make the cash flow projection statement encompass any period of time, but it's a good idea to always have a projection for at least once a month. Enter your estimated revenue for the month.

You'll need to keep a ledger (or use online software) of your expenditures (disbursements). Keep meticulous records of your business's financial activity and you'll be on your way to maintaining a successful – and growing - business.

Financial Strategies

Financial strategies for your business should be a guidebook to financial decisions you'll have to make as your business grows. Just as a good architect plans on a strong foundation before raising the walls, so must you see your financial past before you can plan your financial future.

Treat your Reflexology business like the success it can be. Carefully plan for purchases, expansions, staff and all other matters by looking at the successes (and failures) of the past and then you can concentrate on what's best for the future.

Financial strategy planning can be used like a road map to planning your business success. One of the main problems that keep Reflexologists from developing successful businesses is that they leave out this critical step, content to get by for years to come doing the same things they've done in the past.

This attitude is a passive one and won't get you through the bad times or help your business grow. Anticipating successes and fallbacks (what ifs) can help you deal with any business scenario as it arises.

Here are some points to consider when strategizing your Reflexology business plan:

- Create a budget and stick to it.

- Have a vision and set goals.

- Identify risks associated with your strategic planning.

- Quantify amounts for staff, materials and equipment.

Strategic financial planning in the very beginning stages of your business will ensure that you can diversify and grow when the proper – and most financially strategic – time occurs.

Alternative Health Care is BIG Business

As the baby boomers hit retirement age, health becomes a huge issue. Many boomers will lose their health insurance and others will find that it isn't enough to cover the rising costs associated with medical care.

Millions of boomers and other forward-thinking people are trying alternative medicine as a consideration over traditional medical care. It's not merely the overwhelming costs that are driving the trend – it's also the fact that more information about alternative medicine is becoming available – and, its reputation as a viable option that really works is growing.

The World Health Organization states that Reflexology is considered to be one of the "fastest growing alternative therapies in the world today." It's no wonder that people facing medical concerns should consider Reflexology as an answer to unknown medical concerns for the 21st century.

Boomers, as well as most of the population consider complementary therapies as a way to prevent diseases and practice a healthy lifestyle to remain fit throughout their entire lives. If you've picked NOW as the time to focus on Reflexology as a business that will grow and one in which you can achieve financial success – you've picked the best time.

To the detriment of the profession of Reflexology, some who enter into it don't think of it as a business and formulate a workable business plan. They simply hang out a shingle and charge enough to pay the bills and merely survive – sometimes while working at another job. This can affect the perception of whether Reflexology is a viable way of earning a good living.

That's a shame, because becoming a Reflexologist and opening a business can give you the career and financial security you've always dreamed of. You **can** make over $100,000 per year as a Reflexologist if you're smart about business.

There are specific online courses that will give you a great overview and fill in the blanks with information you didn't know. The are two things to remember: 1. Don't limit yourself. 2. Have a plan in place to achieve the income you deserve.

Steps to Financial Success

The American Reflexology Certification Board offers some valuable suggestions to become financially successful on their website. They include:

You must first become certified as a Reflexologist. "Certification distinguishes the professional from the non-professional, setting apart and bringing credibility to the practitioner who is committed to excellence."

Volunteer. Volunteering is the best way to gain valuable experience in the Reflexology field. Nursing homes, hospitals, high-stress businesses, salons and gyms are just some of the places that might welcome your services – and, some might become clients later on.

Acquire start-up capital. If you don't have a savings for your Reflexology venture, you may want to seek a loan from family or friends or a bank or credit union loan designated for small businesses.

Get a business license. Do your online research and go through the necessary steps to do business in your local area.

Make a decision on where your business location will be. If you want or require minimum output for operating costs, you may want to consider making house calls at least at first. Your home is another option.

Your success depends on your marketing efforts. Use all resources available to let potential clients know that you've opened your business. Have an advertising budget and use it to optimize your output.

Cultivate repeat business. Besides offering quality services to make sure people return, offer them incentives, like discounts and specials on a periodic basis.

Join a mentoring program. There are online programs specifically designed to teach and coach you along the way to a successful Reflexology business. The fee they charge is miniscule compared to the personalized resources that you acquire.

Enhance your education. It's always great to go beyond what you learned in the initial Reflexology training process and learn new techniques that will help your clients – and ensure your financial success.

Act now. Get busy on the dream and vision you have for a successful Reflexology business. Sit down, make a plan and then go about carrying it out.

Now is the time to realize your dreams and make money during the time that alternative health care is growing and thriving. You'll be changing lives for the better – especially yours and your family's – and realize financial success beyond your dreams.

It's Not Just About Money

We've talked a lot in this chapter about making your Reflexology business a financial success – and that's very important. But, it's also important that you consider yourself a professional and worthy of charging fees along the lines that other health care providers charge.

Many Reflexologists are reluctant to call themselves a professional and charge accordingly, but if you've been through the training, set up a business and are confident in your Reflexology skills, you should be confident that you're good enough to call yourself "professional" and charge accordingly.

You'll find that by becoming a professional, you'll get more respect from clients and others in the Reflexology field. You'll also be helping up-and-coming Reflexologists to realize their worth and promote the practice as a health care program that can really help people overcome medical maladies.

Don't wait for another course or another certificate to claim your right to be a professional health care provider. As a Reflexologist, you have remarkable skills and the abilities to heal and relieve pain. Consider yourself a professional and an expert in your field – and others will too.

Chapter 5 - The Future of Reflexology

The great news is that the entrepreneurial future in the health services industry looks bright and promising. As a world population, our health care system must move to the realm of 'prevention' rather than the costly effect of addressing health problems once they occur.

Alternative and complementary health care is part of the new-age model of prevention and maintaining our mental and physical health. Holistic methods are enjoying a surge in popularity and among these rapidly progressing healing arts are massage, acupuncture and Reflexology.

It's become so popular that companies are realizing the importance of these methods to keep employees stress-free and in good health. Food markets have joined the crusade for preventative health measures and are offering healthy and organic foods that aren't processed with harmful preservatives and chemicals.

In a world full of financial fears, job losses and company failures, the health care field has been continuously stable and is one of the only areas where there is fantastic growth potential.

Affordable Holistic Methods

More people are turning to holistic health care than ever before. This result is mainly because of the continuing spiralling high costs of using normal health care methods, but also because people are becoming more aware of the healing powers of holistic medicine.

Therapeutic touch such as Reflexology is being used today to aid the body's natural healing process, recover more rapidly from illnesses, keep the body's immune system healthier and for pain relief.

As people are realizing that this type of therapy gives them better and longer-lasting results and increases their chances of full recovery, they're more likely to try other forms of holistic healing methods.

Reflexology, for example, uses specific touch techniques to rid the body of blockages and congestion around nerve endings that keep the body from healing itself and returning to a balanced state.

Besides trying to escape high medical costs, people are now realizing that holistic medicine is a method that cares for the entire person, including spirit, mind and body. By strengthening the immune system, individuals with chronic medical problems can be cured or at least helped and deadly diseases, such as cancer and heart disease, can be averted.

Differences Between Reflexology & Western Methods

Reflexologists and other holistic healers educate their clients about using the body to heal itself. Generally a Western medicine practitioner seeks to diagnose the disease and then treat it.

When you begin your Reflexology business, you can become highly successful if you can educate your new clients on the different approaches of Eastern vs. Western healing methods.

The participation of the patient is the main difference between the approaches of the two methods. As a Reflexologist, you will engage your clients in the healing process. The Western doctor or MD usually seeks a prescription or surgical procedure to cure the patient – who is passive in the treatments.

Your clients know their bodies better than anyone, and if you can engage them in their own path to good health, they'll recover more quickly and be able to treat themselves – with your guidance.

Holistic medicine isn't a quick fix – it's a journey where the client must take some responsibility for his or her own health. This might mean a lifestyle change such as diet, exercise and meditation. As a holistic practitioner, you can lead them in the right direction.

You can play a big part in your clients' health and wellness and even give them guidance about how to handle an emergency health situation, should it arise. Holistic methods such as Reflexology are safe and they work!

A Window of Opportunity for Reflexologists

The current economic downturn is a direct cause of people reassessing their lives and deciding to leave a "job" and go into business for themselves. We now want independence and the opportunity to give up the nine to five mentality, spend more time with our families and be our own boss.

The economic demise is also an opportunity for making more money than you ever realized was possible.

Statistics reveal that stress is the reason for over 75% of visits to a health care provider. Statistics also report that Reflexology is one of the best methods of relaxation and to relieve the pain and anxiety that stress brings to our lives.

For most of the general population, it comes down to whether you want to take a possibly harmful and addictive pill for stress or turn to a natural method such as Reflexology, meditation, massage and herbal medicine.

Western cultures are finally catching on to what Eastern cultures have known for centuries – that alternative medicine can make a profound and positive difference in our lives.

Baby Boomers & Alternative Health Care

In the year, 2011, the first wave of "notorious" baby boomers turned 65 years old. This event alone brought about an incredible impact on the health care system. Along with age comes the usual aches, pains and diseases, but boomers seem convinced that they can thwart the hands of time and live to a ripe old age without the usual health problems.

Although a single personality can't be attributed to an entire generation, the baby boomers have earned the reputation for wanting self-fulfilment by taking care of themselves and living a good life well into the later years of their lives.

Rather than turning to drugs as the way to live a healthy future life, the majority of boomers are turning to alternative health care methods, including Reflexology. One study states that by the year 2030, "more than six out of ten baby boomers will be managing more than one chronic medical condition." (Source: www.aha.org)

The study also states that over 70% of boomers are now turning to some sort of complementary health care to overcome those conditions. Massage, chiropractor and Reflexology are some of the top alternative choices for boomers.

Hospitals and physicians aren't keeping up with the needs of these aging boomers, which is another reason that alternative medical care is on the rise. Another is the rising cost of traditional health care and loss of insurance benefits.

The "Law of Supply and Demand" dictates that something has to happen to meet the demands of the baby boomers in the future. Alternative treatments seem to be at least part of the answer.

In fact, one article about alternative health care for boomers states that, "Boomers are embracing complementary health care like they've embraced designer reading glasses." What used to be a sign of "old age" is now becoming a chic trend and the boomers are all jumping on the bandwagon.

Health care alternatives such as Reflexology have seen rapid growth in popularity during the last decade

"The bottom line is that Americans spend a lot of money on CAM products, classes, materials and practitioner visits," reported National Center for Complementary and Alternative Medicine (NCCAM) Director Josephine P. Briggs, MD. "We estimate that this (represents) approximately 11% of the total out-of-pocket spending on health care."

Overall out-of-pocket expenditures for complementary and alternative medicines accounted for 1.5% of the $2.2 trillion spent on health care during the year prior to the survey.

Out-of-pocket spending on herbal supplements, chiropractic visits, meditation, and other forms of complementary and alternative medicines (CAM) was estimated at $34 billion in a single year.

One other interesting highlight from the 2007 NCHS and NCAAM report is that in 2007, 38 million adults made an estimated 354 million visits to CAM practitioners, at an estimated cost of almost $12 billion dollars, paying out of their own pockets.

The estimate was based on responses to a national health survey conducted in 2007 by the CDC's National Center for Health Statistics (NCHS).

Previously reported figures based on the same national survey showed that 38% of adults and 12% of children under the age of 18 used some type of alternative medicine in 2007.

The current revolution of alternative medicine, including Reflexology, reflects the boomers' excitement and willingness to explore new methods of treating health problems. It's not only the boomers that are helping expand the knowledge of complementary health care. Technology is also helping to break through old ways of seeing and thinking of the future of medical care.

How to Become a Reflexologist

If you're looking for a safe career and one that's rewarding, both financially and personally, Reflexology is definitely a career that you should look into. First, you must have a thirst for knowledge and a strong desire to help people heal and de-stress their lives.

Basically, Reflexology is a method of applying gentle pressure to specific areas of the feet, hands, ears and face. The nerves in these areas are the entrances into the entire system of the body. If you look at a Reflexology chart, you'll see the labels indicating the nerves that are specific to a certain part of the body.

Reflexology is the miracle stimulator that can stimulate your blood flow and help the organs and the immune system by flushing out harmful toxins that build up in your body. Reflexology methods have been known to help chronic conditions such as sinus, headaches, PMS, insomnia, even fertility problems – and much more.

Specializing in a certain area of Reflexology is a good way to build clientele and get the word out that you're a specialist. For example, if you are great at relieving neck and shoulder pain associated with stress, add that to your brochure or advertising. You may want to include some testimonials from clients who praise your work.

Remember that most people don't really want to know or care about how Reflexology works. They only want to get relief from pain associated with whatever malady they're suffering from.

One of the best ways to decide if a career in Reflexology is best for you is to try it yourself. Talk to successful Reflexologists. Get a treatment and see how you feel afterward. Chances are you'll see right away the reasons why Reflexology is a booming business that's coming on strong in the health industry.

Medical grants are now being issued to study the feasibility of Reflexology treatments – and that's great news for those who want to pursue a career in Reflexology. The grants establish that the safety, efficiency and feasibility of Reflexology are real and that Reflexology can substantially improve a person's ability to walk and breathe better.

Invest in the best training for yourself. Interview colleges and training centres before you decide on which is best for you. You'll want instructors who are tuned in to making a successful business with the skills you'll be learning.

After you choose to pursue Reflexology as a career, you'll likely hear the term 'Complementary Alternative Medicines" (CAM for short). Reflexology is part of the CAM group and considered to be one of the most economic and safest ways to treat certain medical maladies such as headaches, backaches or insomnia.

Healers at Heart

Reflexologists tend to be "healers at heart," and don't often think about the financial side of their business as they're training and setting up a practice. But, making a good living – even making over $100,000 per year is within reach if we think of ourselves as professionals and demand a fair price for our skills.

Reflexology is, and promises to continue to be, one of the top five career choices in holistic health trends. As more people flock to alternative methods of medical care and prevention of diseases – and run from traditional medical care and its high costs, Reflexology will grow by leaps and bounds.

Online classes are available, but be sure and do your research ahead of time to ensure that the instructors and experienced and certified and that the site offers the methods and continuing support that you need. You'll also want to look for a complete course that offers help on the business side of Reflexology.

Look at the practice of Reflexology as more than manipulating feet and hands. You'll do well in business as a Reflexologist if you are educated in biology, chemistry, physiology, ethics and professionalism.

If you can offer other services, such as Facial Reflexology, Meridian Reflexology, Brazilian Toe Massage, or Reading the Feet, your business can increase more rapidly in income and potential. Even if you don't become certified in another area, you can hire "partners" in your business that will boost income and client base.

Work with other Reflexologists who have developed successful businesses and get their input on fees and services they offer. Then you'll have a solid foundation in mind about how to start your own business.

You may want to consider developing a niche with your business. For example, you can spread the word through brochures and advertising that you specialize in relieving neck and back pain.

This can build your business at a good pace right away. And later, if you decide to add other professionals, they can be an extension of you and provide other services.

Be sure that you formulate a plan before hanging your Reflexology shingle. This will ensure that your business flows smoothly in the beginning days and months when you may be too busy to sit down and devote the needed time to it.

The ultimate plan for your Reflexology practice should include a vision statement, a mission statement, and business plan, advertising budget and marketing tools. After you have those items in place, you should be able to open the doors of your business with confidence.

There has never been a better time to invest in your health, the health of your family – the physical health and the financial health. Discover the benefits, the many benefits of foot Reflexology today.

About the Authors

Lauren Slade

Lauren Slade is the Founder and Principal of the Universal College of Reflexology, established since 1991. She is a Past President of the Reflexology Association of Canada and sits on the Advisory Committee for the Natural Therapies Certification Board for Reflexology. Lauren has authored 27 Reflexology manuals for the Universal College of Reflexology's under and post graduate certification and diploma programs. Lauren is a Master Herbalist, with over 35 years' experience in all aspects of Reflexology.

Jack Marriott

Jack Marriott is Co-Principal of the Universal College of Reflexology and currently serves as Vice-President Reflexology with the Natural Therapies Certification Board in the US. He is a past Vice President, Reflexology Association of Canada and a past Vice-President, Reflexology Association of British Columbia. Prior to entering the field of Reflexology and Complementary therapies, Jack was a corporate executive and served as President of the Investment, Commercial and Industrial Division, Real Estate Board of Greater Vancouver in BC Canada and a faculty member of the International Council of Shopping Centres.

Resources

Reflexology Training

Professional Foot Reflexology Practitioner Certification Want to become a Reflexologist and start on the road to earning over $100,000 per year?
http://www.LearnFootReflexologyOnline.com

Reflexology Continuing Education
Already a Reflexologist? Want continuing education credits?
Progressive Reflexology Diploma. Twelve post graduate Reflexology courses: Maternity Reflexology, Facial Reflexology, European Reflexology Techniques, Meridian Reflexology, Reading the Feet, Reflexology and Diabetes, Reflexology and Thyroid Balancing, Reflexology and Allergies, Reflexology and Digestion, Understanding Your Body's Messages, Clinical Reflexology and Banishing Back Pain with Reflexology.
http://www.TheReflexologyZone.com

Reflexology Products

Reflexology Charts, Books available for instant download
http://www.ReflexologyeStore.com

Brazilian Toe Massage is a remarkable drug free therapy that brings a state of calmness and tranquillity to the stressed and hyper-active individual, allowing the body to heal and repair in just minutes. This pressure point massage healing technique with light touches on the toes, as the name suggests, originates from Brazil.   A great add-on service for any Reflexologist, Massage or Wholistic Therapist. Full training Manual (instant download)
http://www.BrazilianToeMassage.com

Reflexology Information

Universal College of Reflexology
http://www.iReflexology.com   &
http://www.ProReflexology.com

Jack Marriott's blog
http://www.JackMarriott.com

Lauren Slade's blog
http://www.LaurenSlade.com

Business and Website Solutions

Expert affordable website solutions for Reflexologists and Wholistic Health Practitioners.

http://www.laurenrecommends.com/websites

Business Success Coaching Successful entrepreneurs understand that, to continue running a business, you can never stop learning. Discover ways to hone your skills and find new success strategies to take your business to the next level.

http://www.laurenrecommends.com/BusinessSuccess

Facebook Business Consulting More than 2.5 million websites are integrated with Facebook and if you are not using this to connect to new customers, you are losing out on potential clients.

http://www.laurenrecommends.com/socialmedia

Index

23936896R00054

Made in the USA
Middletown, DE
08 September 2015